Re|Mindful

Food and Mood Journal.

"A Guide to Authentic Eating"

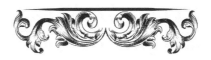

Mindful|Maiden

Re|Mindful

Mindful|Maiden   2

There's always
a new meal."

— Collin McShirley"

Re|**Mindful**

Purpose

The purpose of this guide is to help you examine the reasons why you're overeating. It will help you examine the "why" "what" "when" and "how" of your eating.

Once you start to see a pattern of feelings connected to overeating, you're able to pin point the root of the reason for overeating. This book is most useful when paired with my book "How I Broke Free From Dieting." It shares examples of common reasons why people overeat and how to change negative coping mechanisms into positive coping mechanisms.

Once you identify what is eating you inside it's incredibly helpful to have support. If you're interested in working with me individually, I will provide 24-7 support to examine the feelings at hand that lead to overeating.

Use this journal daily to keep on track. If you miss a few days, it's okay. I always want you to be kind to yourself. There is no right or wrong here. All I ask is that you keep trying and always love yourself in the process.

If you would like to reach out to me, I am available at www.collinmcshirley.com

Re|**Mindful**

About Me

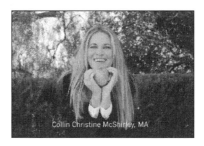

My name is Collin Christine McShirley. I ate emotionally for many years. I didn't always know I was an emotional eater until I received training to be able to identify it. I have a master's degree in clinical psychology and am certified by the Centre for Eating and Dieting Disorders, and Healthy Aging from Boston University.

I believe love heals. Learning to love myself and examining the reasons behind why I was overeating is what helped me heal. I know how you feel because I have personally been there. My goal is to provide the love, support, education, and structure you need so that you can love and support yourself.

If you're interested in learning more about my Authentic Eating Program, Please visit my website at www.collinmcshirley.com

Re|Mindful

Explanation

This book is about you. Look at it as your own personal journal to help you keep track of how you're eating, what you're eating, why you're eating, and when you're eating. This journal helps you identify patterns that you might not see every day without keeping them documented.

Use this journal by reading the daily inspirational quote I provide, or feel free to write your own. Use the Remindful Questions on the next page as guide for every meal.

For every meal, write down the questions provided in the blank space of paper. I personally have 6 well-balanced meals a day, every 3-4 hours as suggested by my dietician. It is important that you work with a professional to determine your dietary needs.

Note: It's best to have a snack in between main meals.

  ❖ Breakfast
  ❖ Snack
  ❖ Lunch
  ❖ Snack
  ❖ Dinner
  ❖ Snack

Every time you go to eat make sure you use these questions as a guide to tune into your eating habits.

Re|Mindful

When I first started this process, it was quite challenging for me to do the work. It was overwhelming not only to fill in the answers to the questions, prepare the meals, and examine the reasons why I was eating, but I also wasn't used to putting so much work into something for the purpose of helping myself. If you've never used a food or mood journal then I would expect you might have the same experience. This is normal. Rome wasn't built in a day.

All you can do is keep trying. I started by filling it out with just breakfast and got comfortable with that, then added snack, lunch, snack, dinner, you get the picture. Don't be overwhelmed by this because you can't mess up. There is no right and wrong here. There is always a new meal and there is always a new moment to fill out your Remindful Journal in order to stay connected to your food and your mood.

Re|Mindful

Remindful Questions

❖ What did you eat?

❖ Are you physically hungry?

❖ Are you distracted while eating?

❖ Where are you?

❖ What do you notice around you?

❖ What are you thinking?

❖ How would you describe your mood?

❖ How much did you eat?

❖ If you felt you overate, what mood did you feel?

❖ If you overate, did you tell yourself there is always a new meal?

Note: Feel free to add your own questions and quotes that inspire you to be an "Authentic Eater."

Re|**Mindful**

Now is always the
time to start being an
authentic eater.

– Collin Christine

Re|Mindful

*Today I will show myself a little more
kindness and a little less judgment.*

Re|Mindful

Today I will try to create something positive in my life. I will create it with love. Music, art, dance, anything you feel like creating.

Re|Mindful

I will write four things I love about what I see in my room.

Re|**Mindful**

I will write four things about what I love about nature.

Re|**Mindful**

I will write four things about what I love about myself.

Re|**Mindful**

I realize that my relationship to food
is life long. I will befriend my body.

Re|Mindful

I will not restrict myself, instead I will feed myself foods that nourish my body and soul.

Re|Mindful

Today I will practice a change
in perspective. If I feel shame after
overeating, it is okay and there is always
a new meal.

Re|Mindful

You're a unique gift who is worthy of love.

Re|Mindful

'Today I choose to be present'. In each moment with every meal.

Re|**Mindful**

Today I will go outside and sit outside for five minutes and breathe.

Re|Mindful

Today I will break the habit of speaking negatively about myself. I will try my best to do so.

Re|Mindful

Yes, I have had many bumps in the road with food but today is a new day. A new start.

Re|**Mindful**

I am learning to stop caring about what others think about me and my body. I am learning to love my body.

Re|Mindful

I am strong because I keep trying.

Re|**Mindful**

Dear Self, thank you for trying your hardest to be the best version of yourself possible. Love, Me

Re|Mindful

*Today I am working on being everything
I need to be happy, healthy, and strong.*

Re|Mindful

There is always a new mew', a new way
to be mindful, and new words to speak
kindly to yourself.

Re|**Mindful**

Think positive thoughts. You can even sing them.

Re|Mindful

There is always a new way to look at something.

Re|**Mindful**

*Happiness is always an inside job,
remember that.*

Re|Mindful

I am starting to love me. Self-love isn't selfish.

Re|Mindful

Vent below.

Re|Mindful

Accept yourself, love yourself, be yourself.

Mindful|Maiden   33

Re|Mindful

I am blessed with all of the love I can provide to myself.

Re|Mindful

Remember, be patient with yourself.
Love yourself through the process.

Mindful|**Maiden**

Re|Mindful

Be your own best buddy.

Re|Mindful

Flowers have to grow through dirt.
Make your way through the soil.

Re|Mindful

How lucky we are to have this very moment, right now, this very second, at peace.

Re|Mindful

Please hug your dark, she needs your light.

Re|Mindful

Let's sigh in relief together, ahhhh I never have to diet again!

Re|Mindful

I am learning to love this incredible body.

Re|**Mindful**

Take your pleasure seriously.

Re|**Mindful**

Do more of what makes you naturally smile.

Re|Mindful

Feed your body the nutrients it needs, say with me now.... "No more restriction. Emotionally, or physically."

Re|Mindful

One day you will wake up and say, " I don't want to fight my body anymore."

Re|Mindful

Hold your heart with warm loving hands.

Re|**Mindful**

Feed your body loving nutrients.

Re|**Mindful**

Our journey with food is life long.
Let's befriend it now.

Re|Mindful

Nothing in nature grows instantly. Give
yourself the proper nutrients to bloom.

Re|Mindful

Make your own path to peace.

Re|Mindful

What we want in life we first must create. Use your imagination. What do you see for yourself?

Re|Mindful

Surround yourself with people who love you and respect you.

Re|Mindful

When we allow the truth in our lives we will start to feed ourselves better nutrients.

Re|Mindful

Promote what you love about yourself daily. Write it, sing it, dance it out!

Re|Mindful

Listen to the rhythm of your progress.
Dance to the beat.

Re|Mindful

A few nice words a day will make life long changes.

Re|**Mindful**

Focus on the present. Happiness isn't a destination it is a process.

Re|Mindful

Accept that where you are right now is perfect. Keep moving forward.

Re|Mindful

Stay focused on all of the things you have in your life to be grateful for.

Re|Mindful

May there always be an authentic eater by your side. If you don't have one in your life, become one.

Re|**Mindful**

You're capable of such amazing things.
Keep walking this path.

Re|**Mindful**

Never tell yourself that you're not good enough.

Re|Mindful

Break free from the chains you put on yourself. You have the support to fly free.

Re|Mindful

Attention provided to yourself is never wasted energy.

Re|**Mindful**

Negative thinking can lead to negative action. If a negative thought comes up and you want to overeat, be kind to yourself and say, "this thought isn't negative I am stressed and I am feeding my body. There is always a new meal."

Re|**Mindful**

Become friends with failure.

Re|Mindful

Please don't feed your tears. If you
do, feed them something that gives you
strength.

Re|Mindful

I will help you rise strong. I am here for you in heart and soul.

Re|Mindful

Start somewhere. Take that first step.
Support is here.

Re|Mindful

We must heal our minds along with our bodies.

Re|**Mindful**

Lighten up. You will start to mentally and physically feel lighter.

Re|Mindful

Learning is exercise for the brain. The more you learn the stronger your brain becomes and you will be able to stay on top of all of the things you want to accomplish.

Re|**Mindful**

When you hold back your voice and your feelings, you're overeating mentally.

Re|**Mindful**

You don't need to change your body to love your body. You can start loving your body right now, just as it is.

Re|Mindful

Food is meant to nourish you. Nourish yourself with foods that make you feel good.

Re|Mindful

Who are you as an eater? What you eat is part of figuring out this story.

Re|Mindful

If you feel you need stability to feel grounded, plant your feet on the ground, put your back against a wall, sit, breathe, and imagine something that you find pleasant.

Re|Mindful

Stop fighting your appetite. Restricting leads to overeating. Welcome your appetite, listen to it, greet it with love when it enters.

Re|**Mindful**

Love is an underrated nutrient.

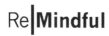

Mindful|**Maiden**

Re|Mindful

When you start to love food, it will magically love you just as much!

Re|Mindful

Breathing in and out while listening to peaceful music always makes me feel lighter inside and out.

Re|Mindful

Trust that there is a light at the end of the tunnel. Just keep driving and keep putting gas in the car by nourishing yourself with food so you can reach your destination.

Re|**Mindful**

Increase your metabolism with the love and laughter you provide yourself!

Re|Mindful

Are you willing to be flexible with what you eat? Flexibility is key to changing your mindset.

Re|Mindful

We are learning as we go along. Day by day, we are kind to ourselves and allowing ourselves to grow.

Re|Mindful

Peace be with food.

Re|Mindful

Self care isn't selfish. You deserve it.

Re|Mindful

You're all that you need. You're beautiful, lovable, and worth your time.

Re|**Mindful**

Live like no one is watching, dance like no one is watching, love like no one is watching, set yourself free.

Re|Mindful

Step by step. Day to day. Moment to moment. Meal to meal. Thought to thought.

Re|**Mindful**

Bring your heart everywhere you go. It is your most trusted advisor.

Mindful|**Maiden**

Re|Mindful

When you find it hard to trust yourself, trust nature, or someone else you truly trust. Trust the consistency of how a river flows.

Re|**Mindful**

Rise each morning. Write four things that you're grateful for.

Re|Mindful

Feel, my friend. Breathe and feel.

Re|Mindful

And if I ask you to name all the things
that you love, how long would it take
to name yourself? - unknown

Re|Mindful

Everyday is a new day to start over.

Re|**Mindful**

Always show kindness to yourself even if you didn't grow up with kindness.

Re|Mindful

Stop comparing yourself to others.
You don't know the path that they walk.
Focus on yourself and all the beauty
you have within.

Re|Mindful

Try and forget about a past that dissatisfies you. Focus on the present. Give yourself the gift to imagine a life that you want, that you believe in.

Re|Mindful

You deserve all the love and light in the world. Open your heart and let it in!

Mindful|**Maiden**

Re|**Mindful**

Take a leap of joy. Build your wings, fly!

Re|Mindful

You can have a fresh start at any moment. You live in the present. This is a gift. Open your eyes to right now. It doesn't matter what happened in the past. You create the present.

Re|Mindful

Do you love animal's? Imagine yourself
as one running free with nature
providing you strength. Trust the earth
beneath you.

Re|Mindful

Do what you can, right now in this moment. Whatever it is, that is enough. It is enough.

Re|**Mindful**

Small steps lead to life long changes.
You can't build your castle over night.

Mindful|**Maiden**   105

Re|**Mindful**

Love food that loves you back.

Re|Mindful

"ReMindful Food and Mood Journal – A guide to Authentic Eating"
Written by Collin Christine McShirley *Copyright © 2016, by Collin Christine McShirley - Published and distributed in the United States by: Collin Christine McShirley. www.CollinMcShirley.com*

Legal

Disclaimer

It is important to remember that everything is this book is based on true stories, actual events and living people. Some names of some characters have been changed simply to follow legal and privacy protocols. From time to time I do use names that are in the public domain. For everyone, I invite you to use your own experiences, imagination, and visualize the people in your life who fit the events I use to create the unique Authentic Eating Program TM for us. The value in this book exists in learning, distinguishing and personally owning the Authentic Eating Program TM distinctions available from these stories for yourself and in your life with others. Authentic Eating Program TM distinctions are the Gold for you and your life. The actual who, what, and where are the entertainment elements that bring life to being a Authentic Eating Program TM under any circumstance. An irony of life will always be that "non-fiction is based on fiction." My truths may or may not match your truths, but both will always create ways of living life. Focus on the Authentic Eating Program TM distinctions in your life; what is truth will exist in actions, whether it is fiction disguised as non-fiction or not.

ISBN-13: 978-1523479719
ISBN-10: 152347971X (CreateSpace Assigned ISBN.)

Re|Mindful

Made in the USA
San Bernardino, CA
23 November 2018